I love Yummy Fruits!

Fruits give me energy to run, play and learn.

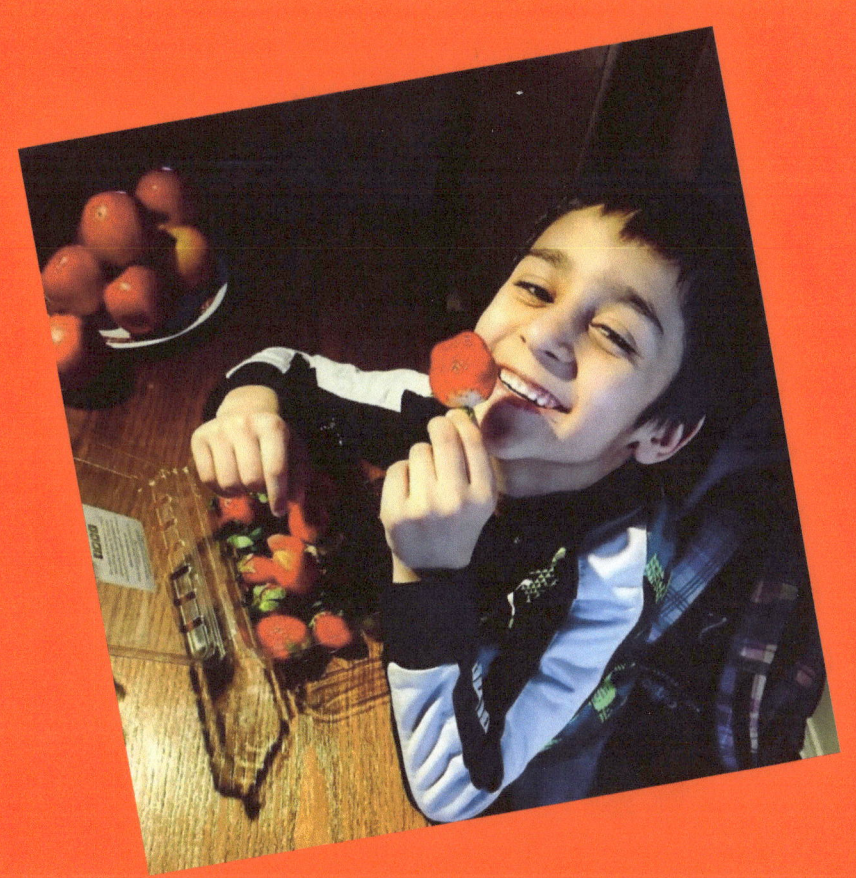

Fruits A to Z
Alphabetical order

Written by Nabila Kiyani

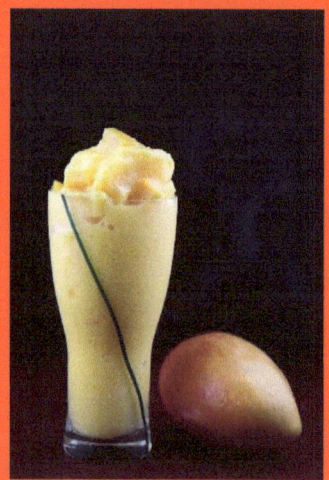

This book belongs to……………………

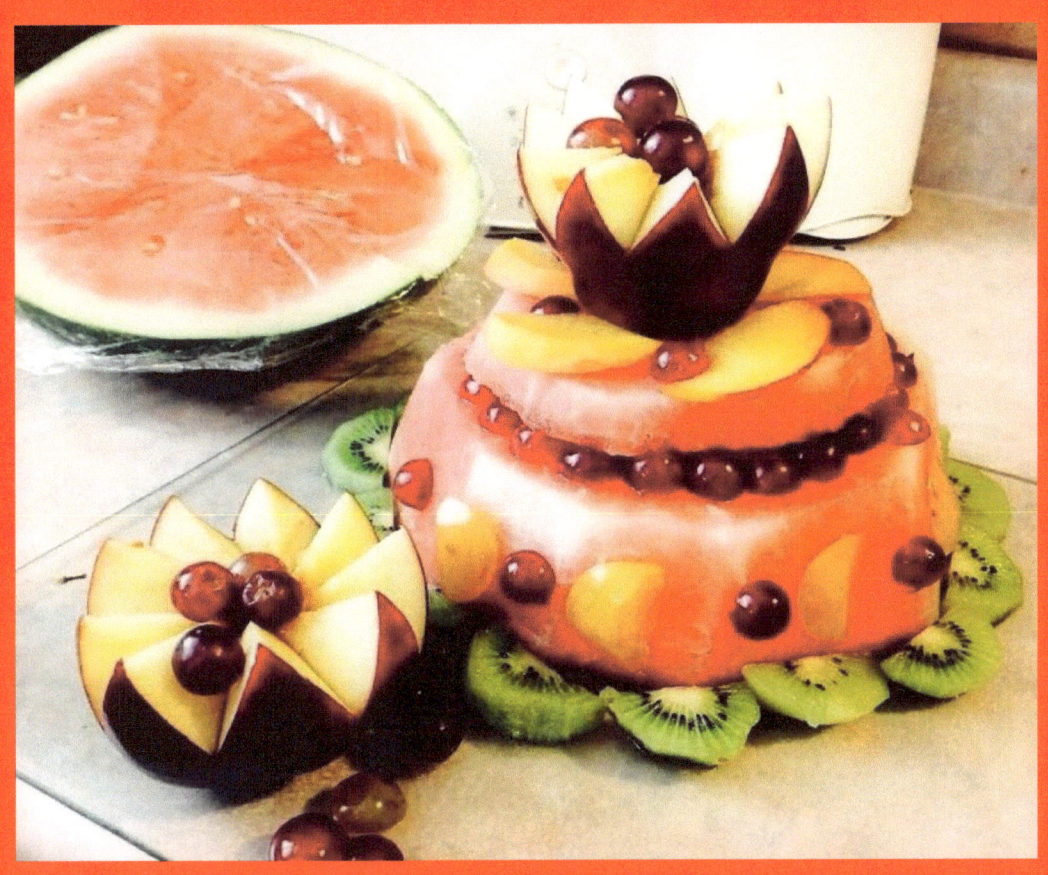

I love Yummy Fruits!

Fruits give me energy to run, play and learn!

Nabila Kiyani

ISBN-13: 978-1544730363 Printed in the United States of America

ISBN-13: 978-1544730363

DEDICATION

I dedicate this book to children around the world. Living a healthy lifestyle starts from the early years. I encourage all of you to read fruits and vegetable books to children. Every sale of this book will help the poor, needy, and homeless.
Thank You for your support!

ACKNOWLEDGMENTS

This book was inspired by my Parents, Family, Teachers and my experience at the Institute for Integrative Nutrition® (IIN), where I received my training in holistic wellness and health coaching. IIN offers a truly comprehensive Health Coach Training Program that invites students to deeply explore the things that are most nourishing to them. From the physical aspects of nutrition and eating wholesome foods that work best for each individual person, to the concept of Primary Food – the idea that everything in life, including our spirituality, career, relationships, and fitness contributes to our inner and outer health – IIN helped me reach optimal health and balance. This inner journey unleashed the passion that compels me to share what I've learned and inspire others. Beyond personal health, IIN offers training in health coaching, as well as business and marketing. Students who choose to pursue this field professionally complete the program equipped with the communication skills and branding knowledge they need to create a fulfilling career encouraging and supporting others in reaching their own health goals. From renowned wellness experts as Visiting Teachers to the convenience of their online learning platform, this school has changed my life, and I believe it will do the same for you. I invite you to learn more about the Institute for Integrative Nutrition and explore how the Health Coach Training Program can help you transform your life. Feel free to contact me to hear more about my personal experience at [www.nabilakiyani.com], or call (647) 767-5033.

I Love Yummy Fruits!

Written by Nabila Kiyani

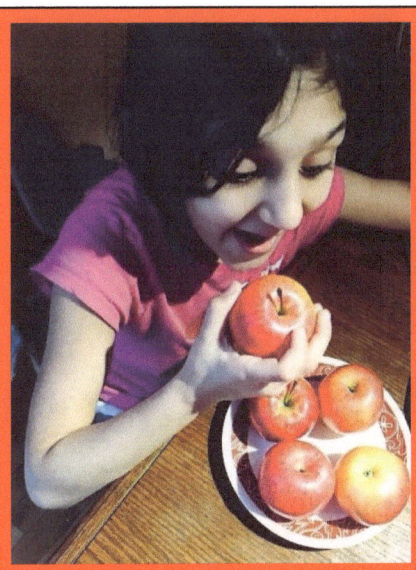

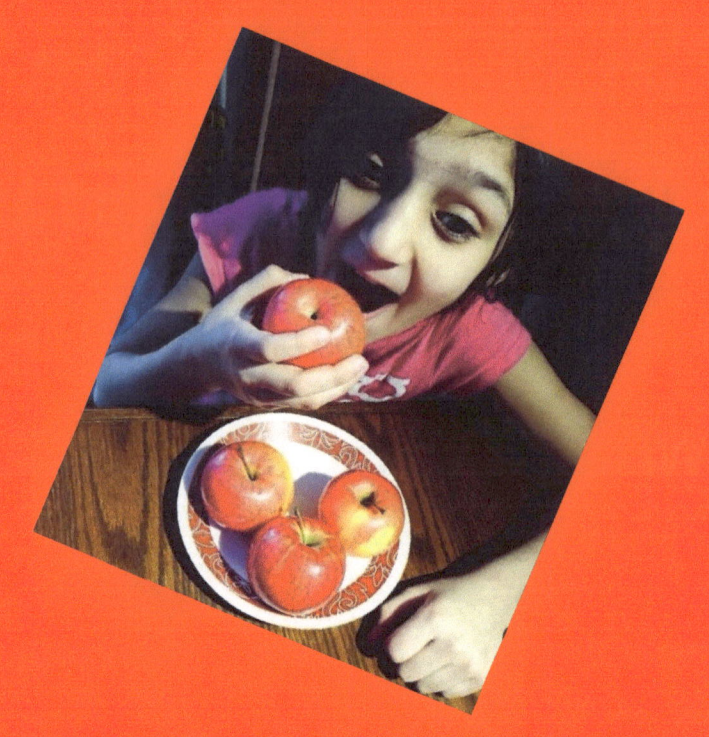

I love to eat Apples.

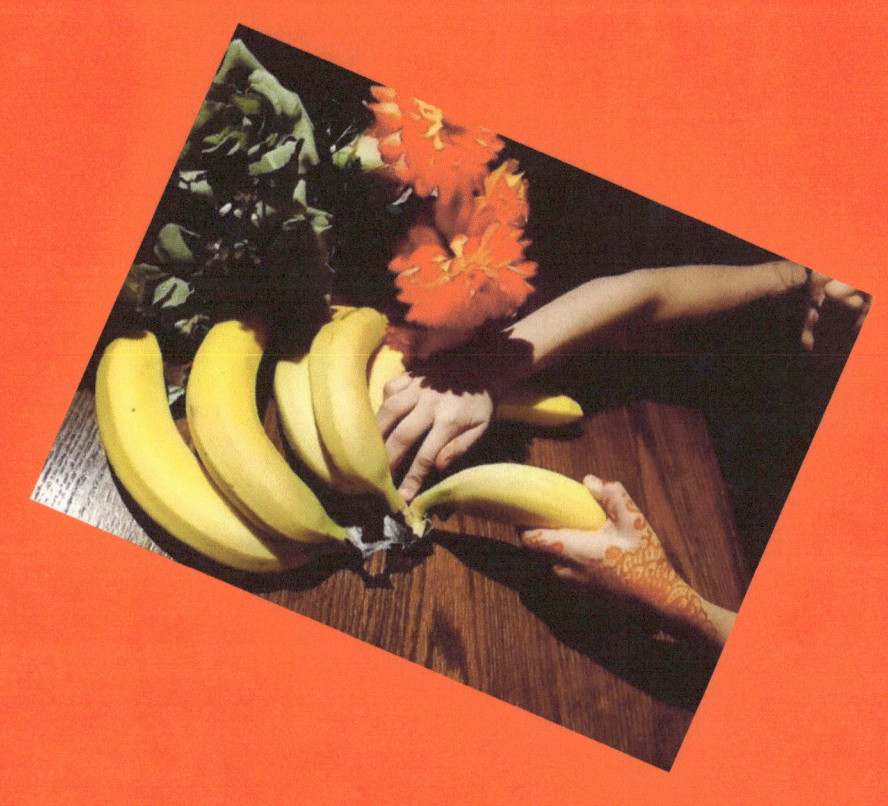

I love to eat Banana and
Banana Smoothie....

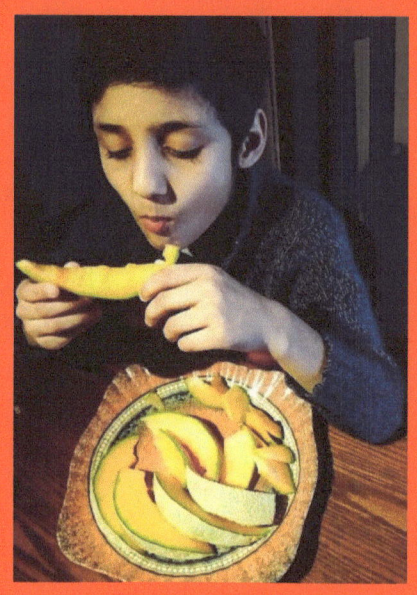

I love to eat Cantaloupe.

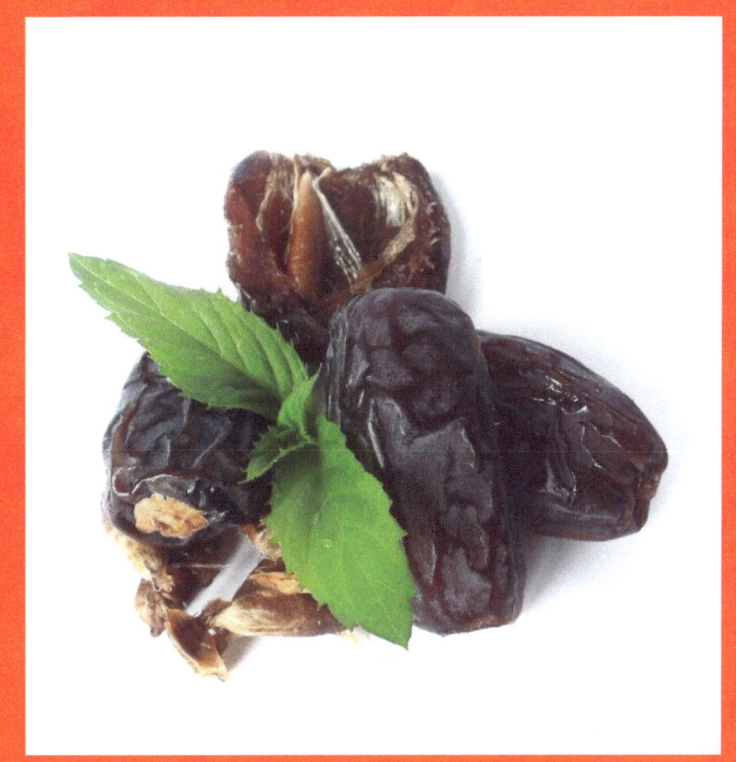

I love to eat Dates.

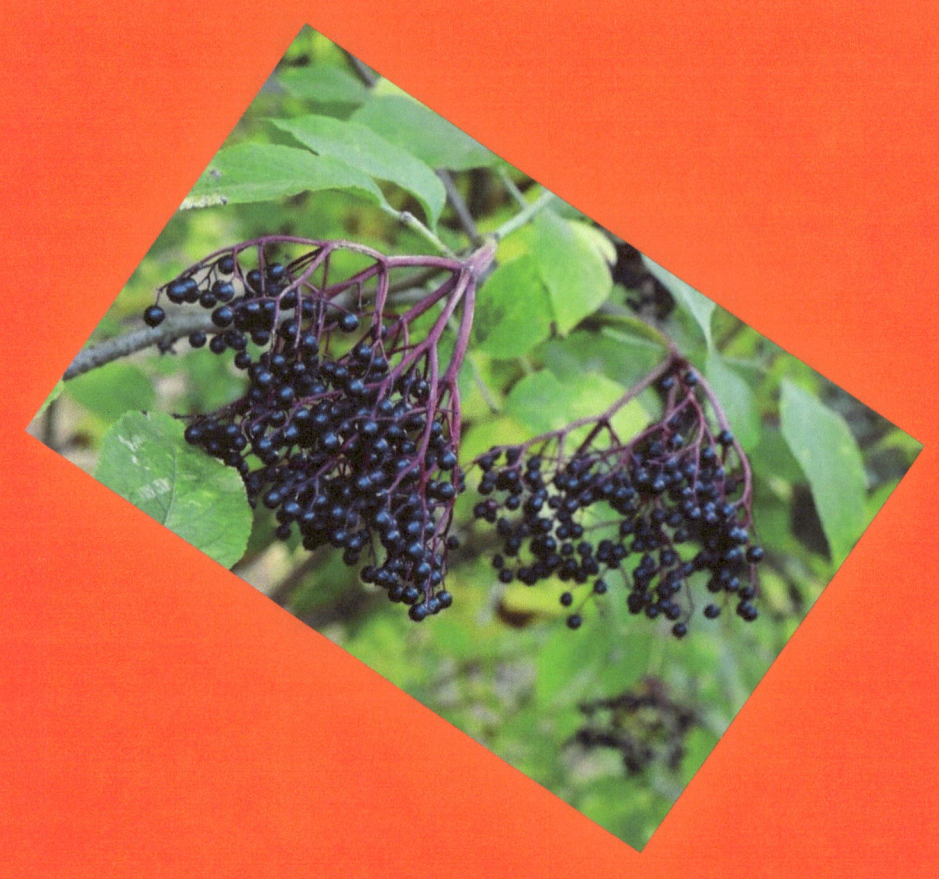

This is Elderberry.

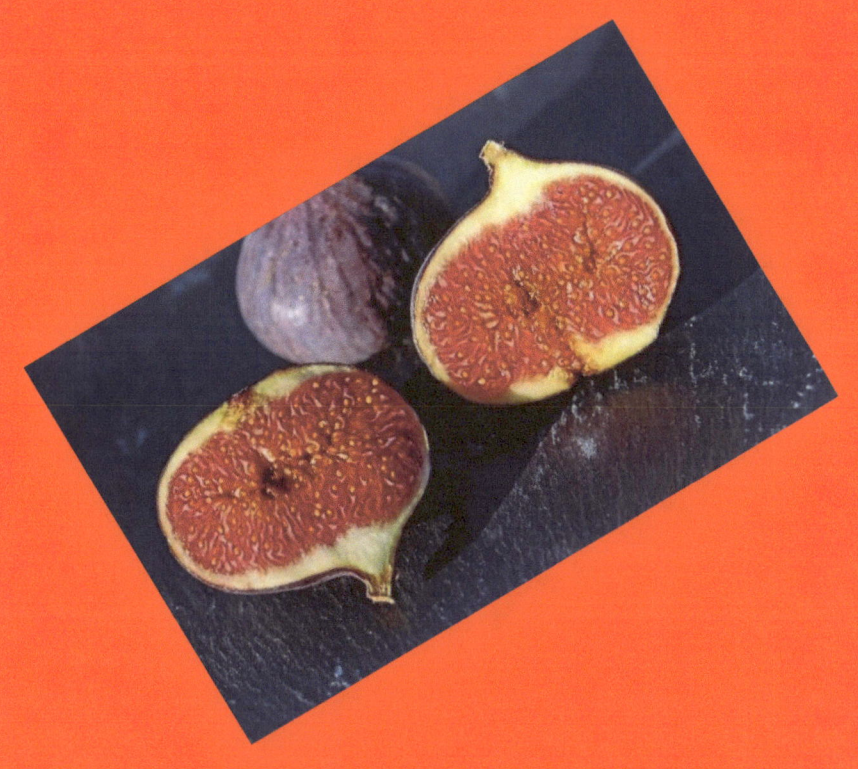

I love to eat Figs.

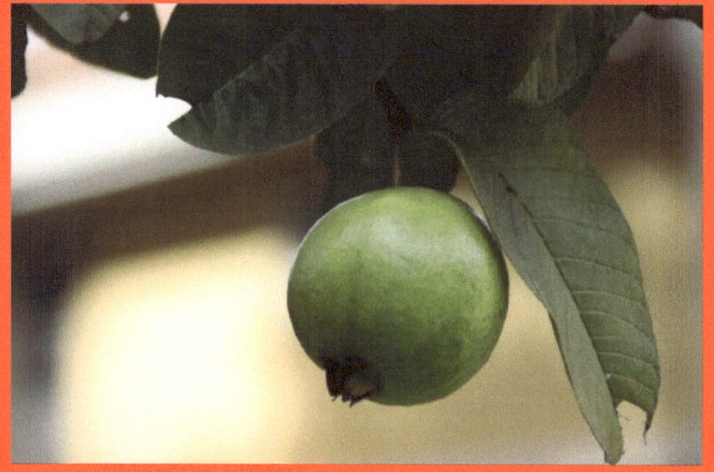

I love to eat Guava.

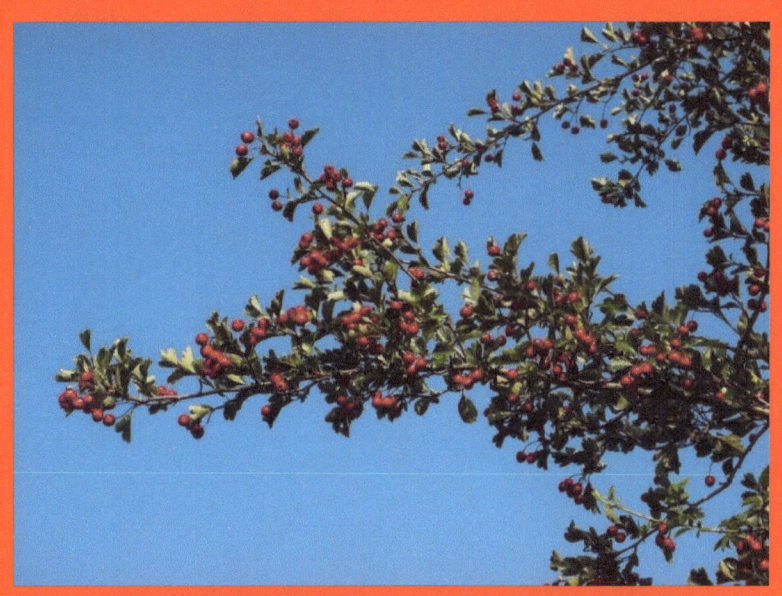

This is Hawthorn fruit...

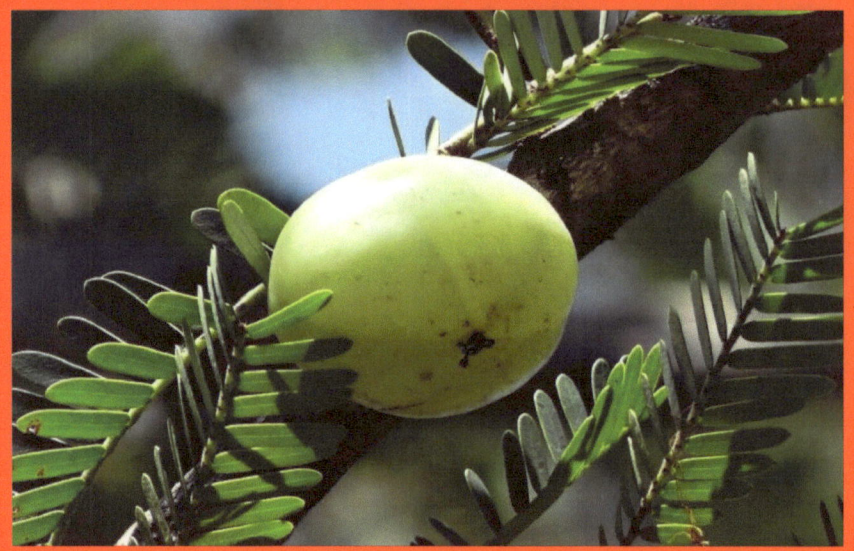

.... And an Indian Gooseberry.

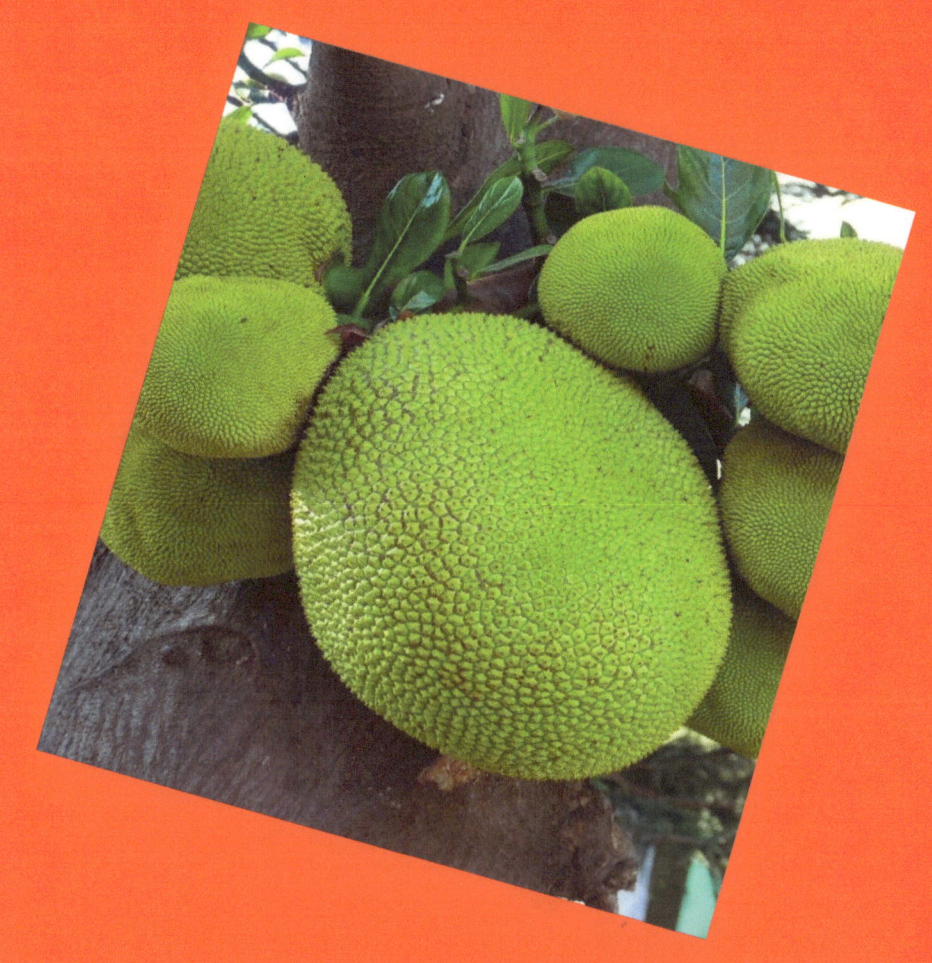

I love to eat Jackfruit.

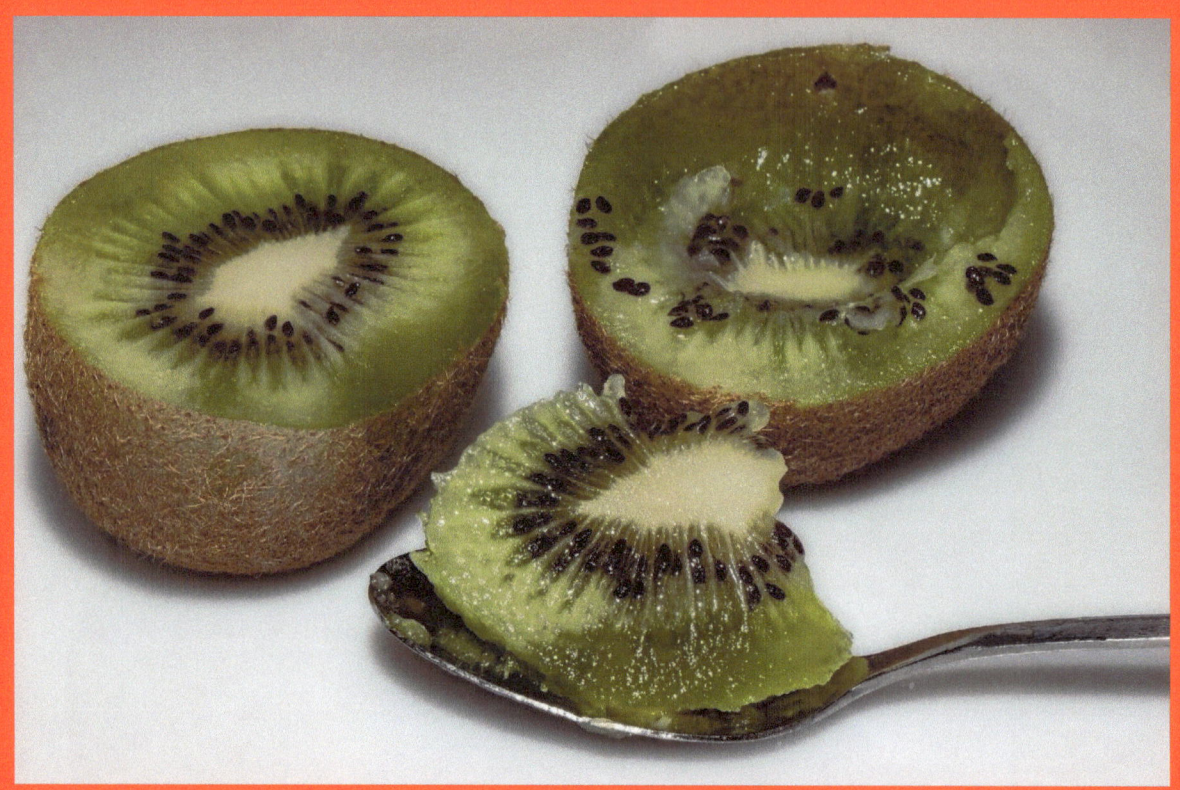

I love to eat Kiwi.

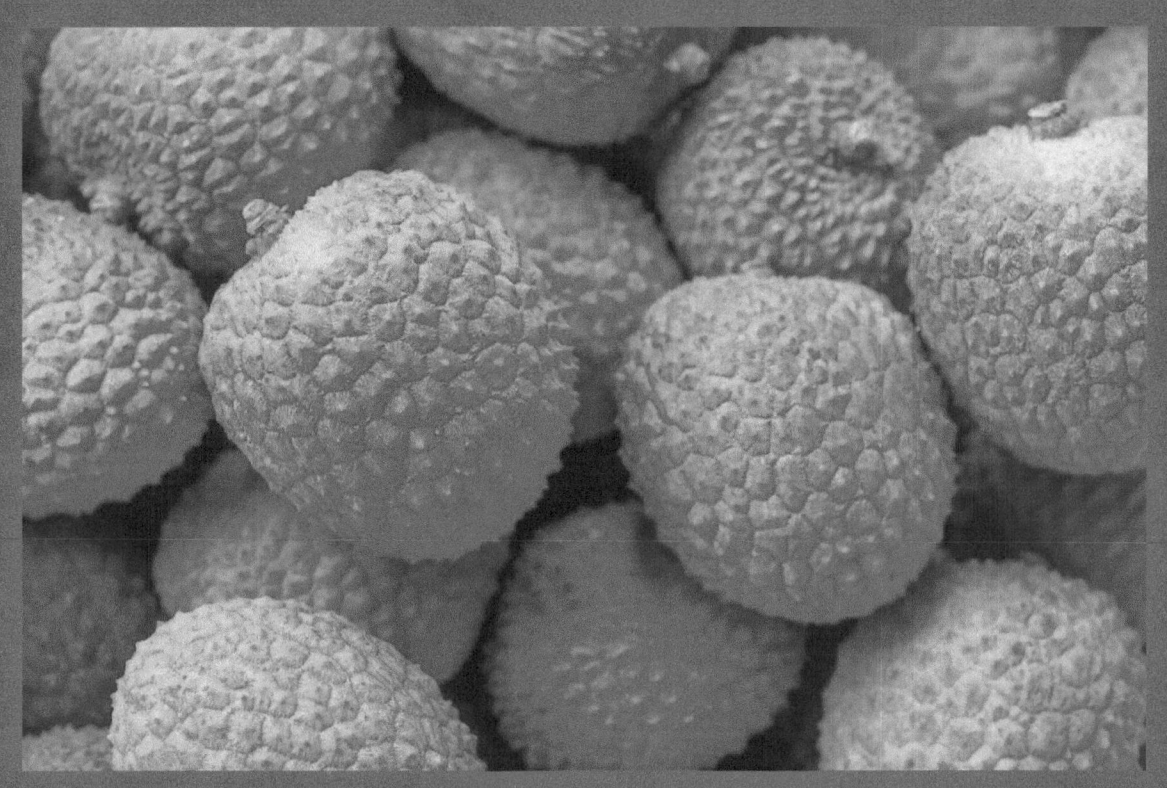

I love to eat Lychee.

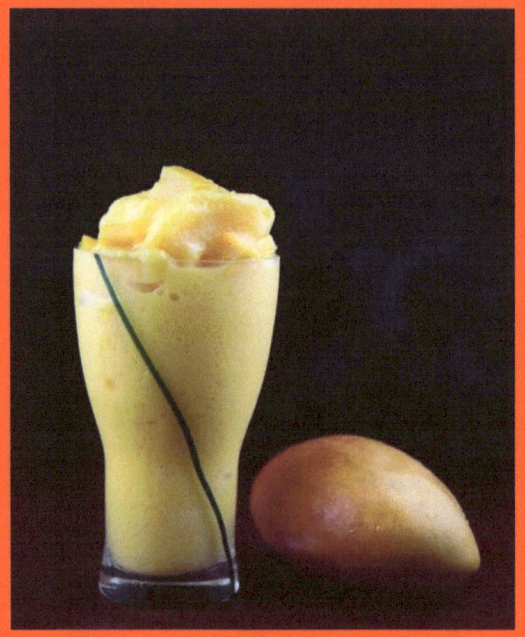

I love Mango Smoothie

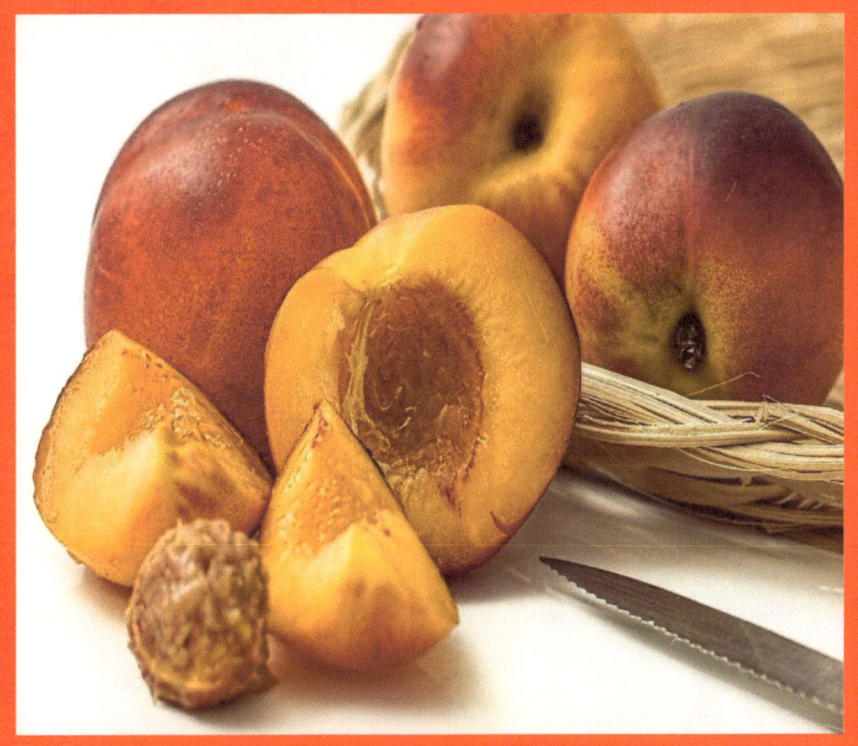

I love to eat Nectarines.

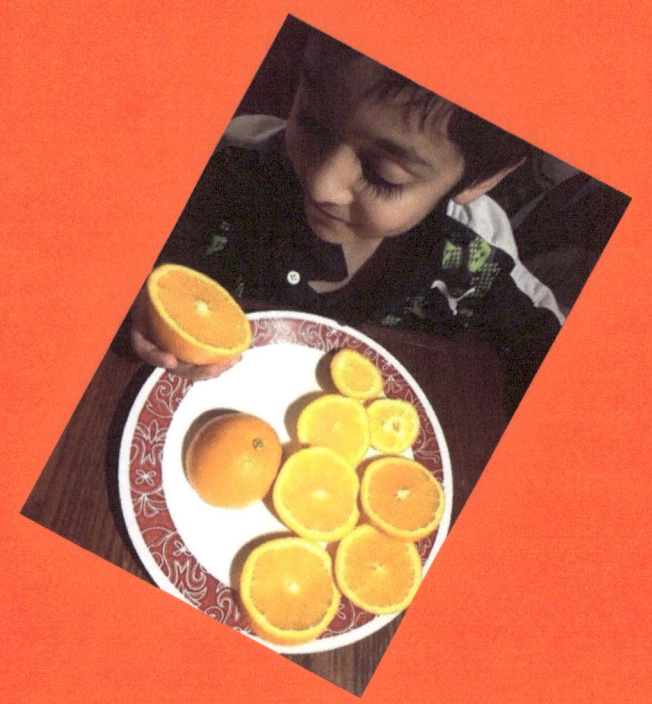

I love to eat Oranges.

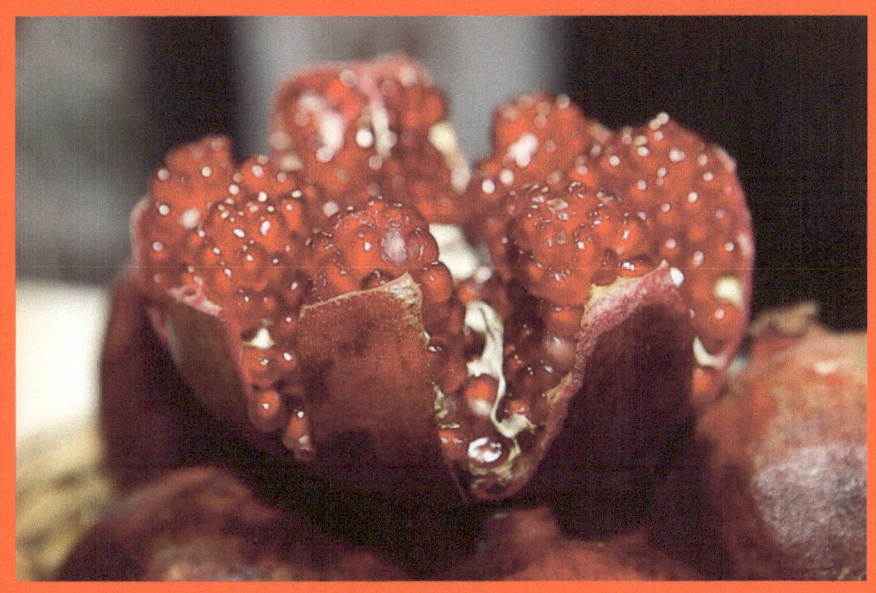

I love to eat Pomegranate.

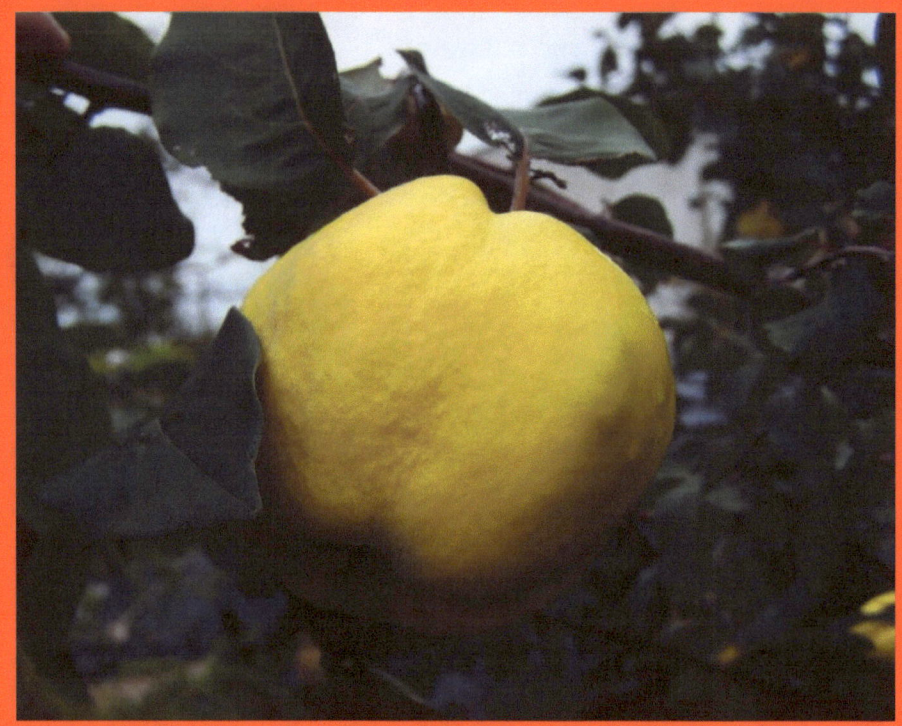

This is a Quince fruit.

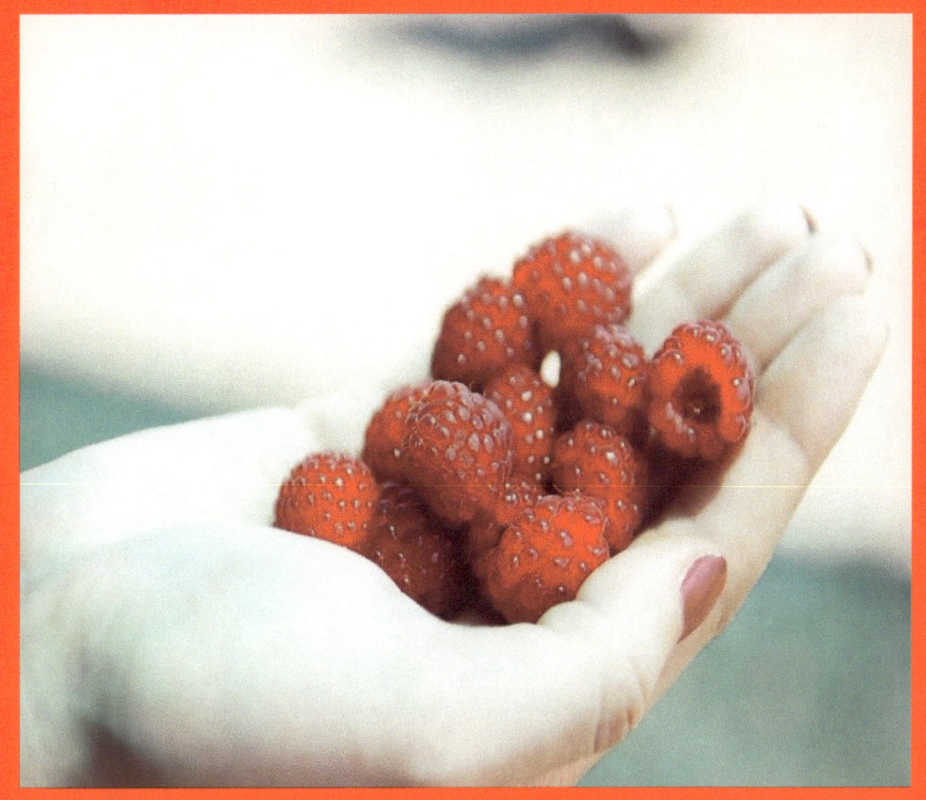

I love to eat Raspberries.

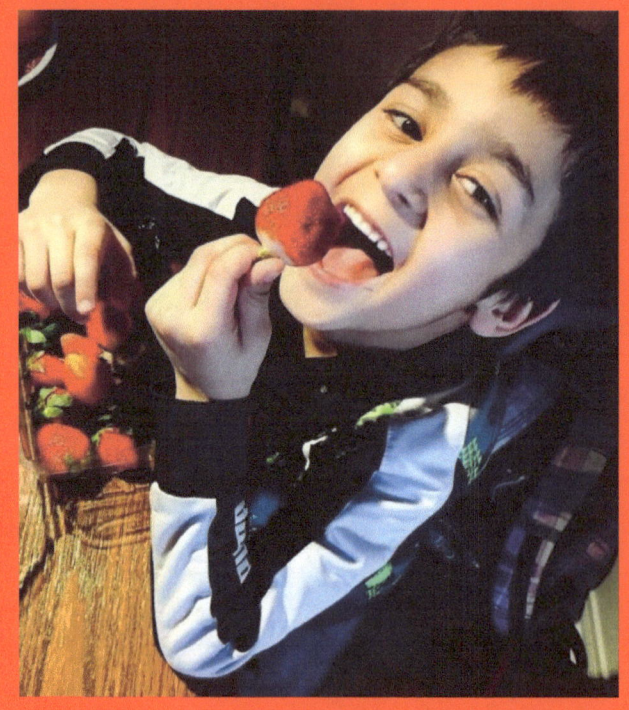

I love to eat Strawberries.

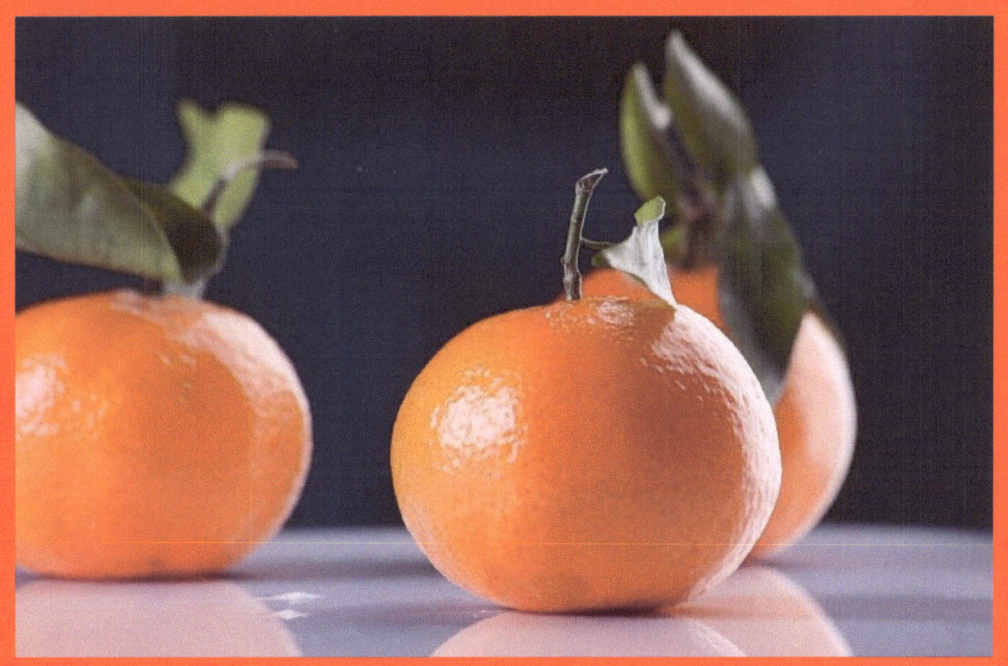

I love to eat Tangerines.

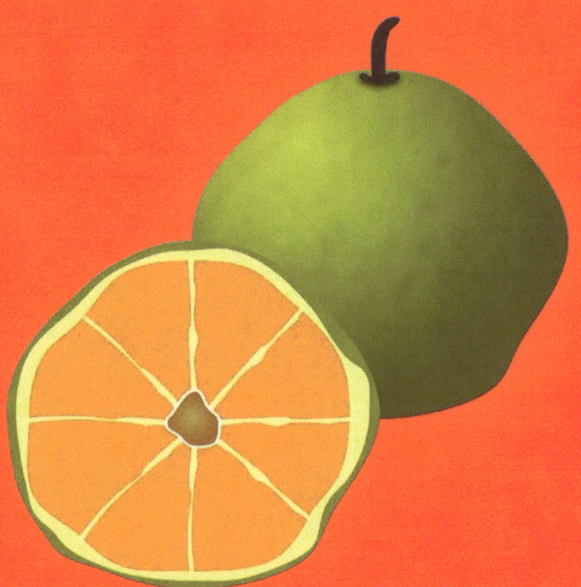

This is Ugli fruit.

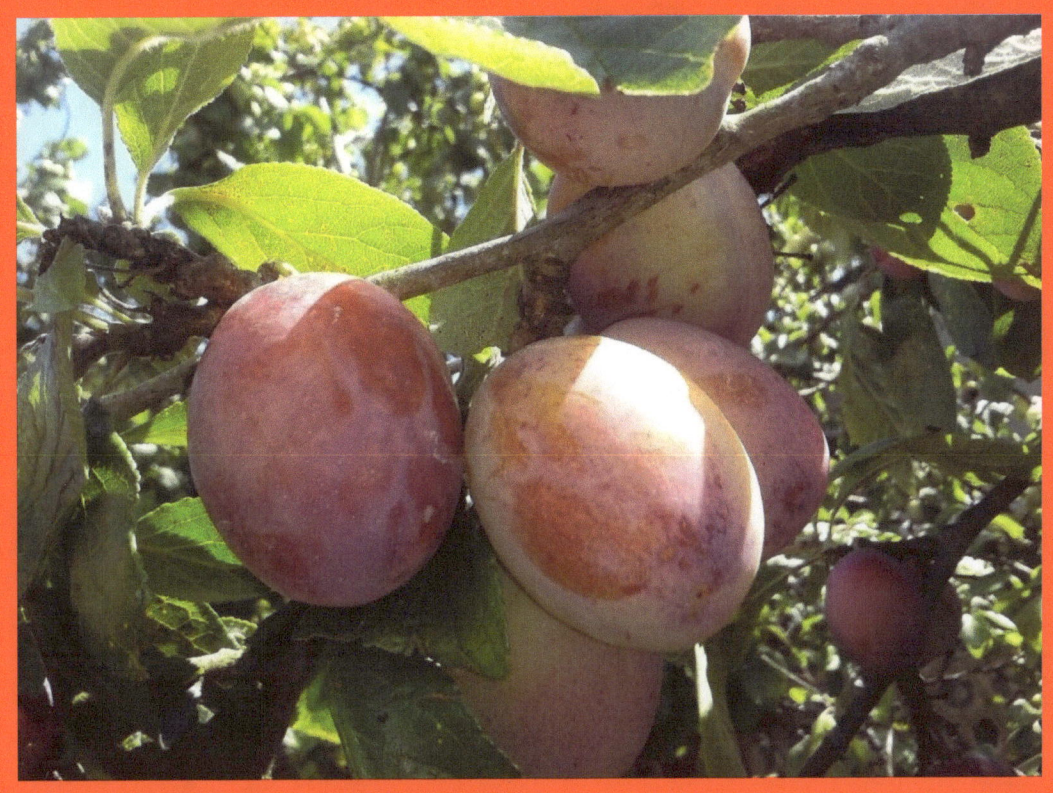

....and Victoria plum.

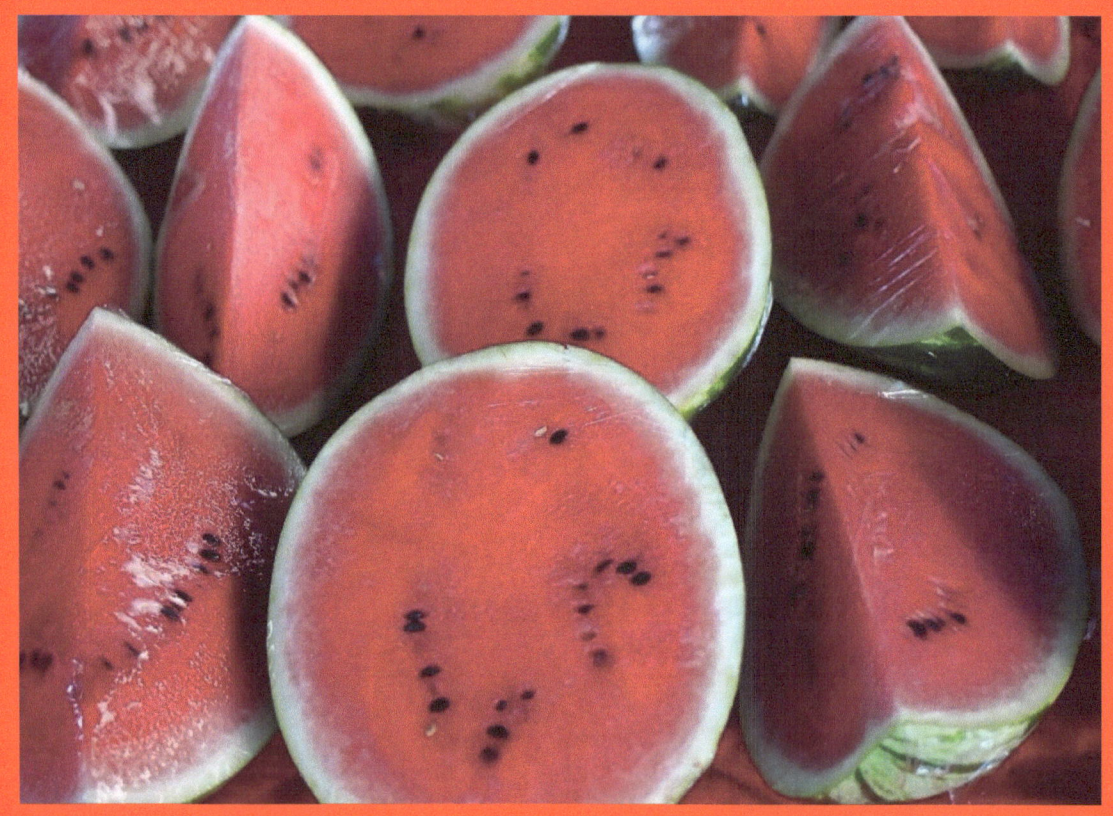

I love to eat Watermelon and Watermelon Juice Yummmmm……

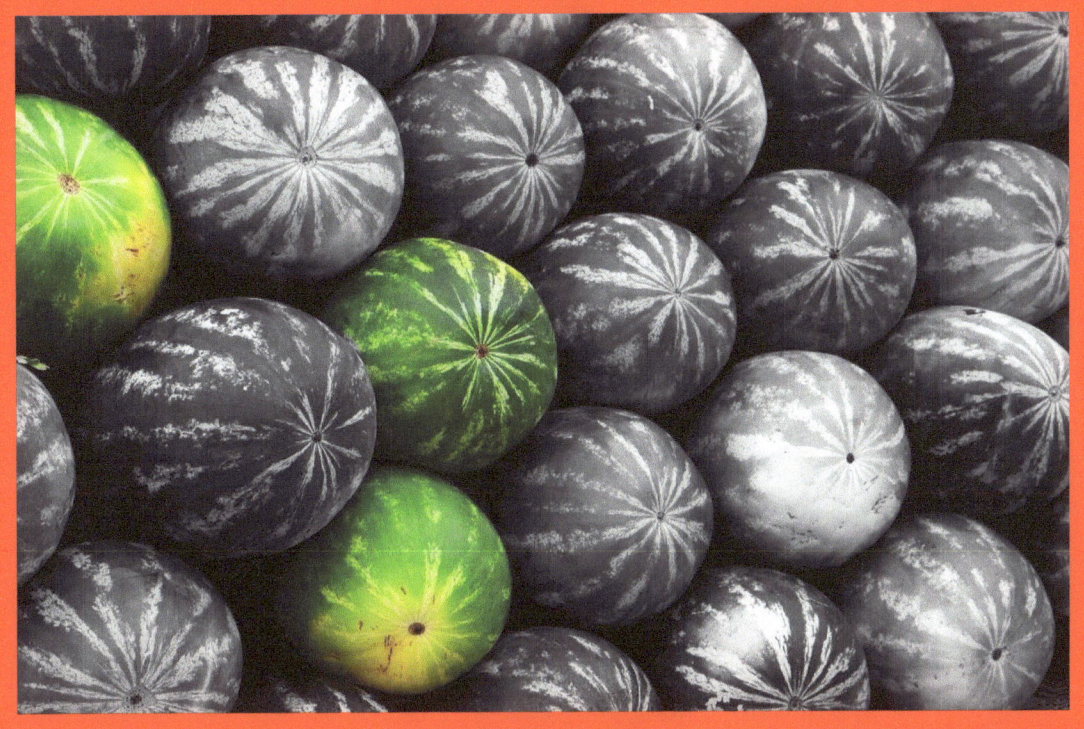

This is Xigua. It is Chinese Watermelon black from outside and red from inside. ....hmmm......

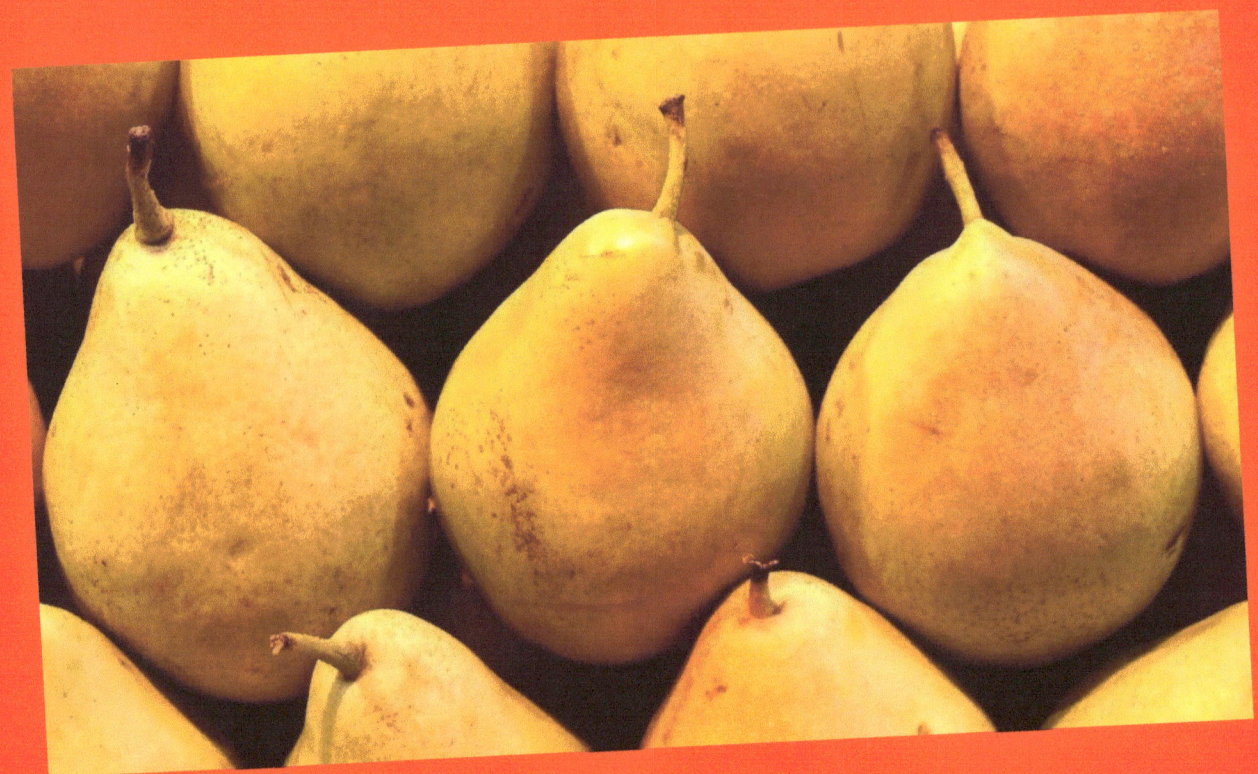

This is Yali Pear.

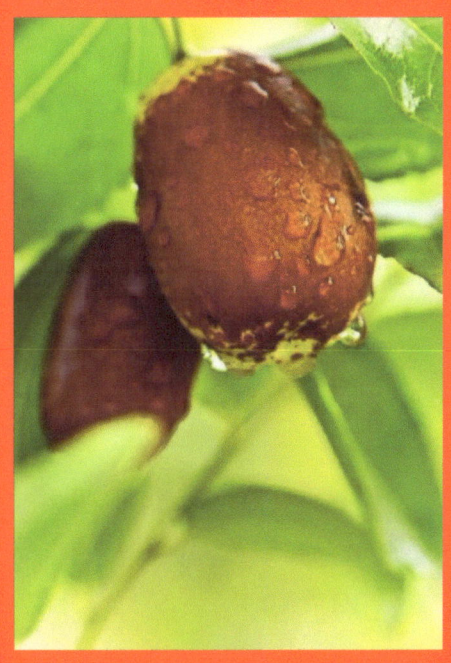

....and Ziziphus Jujuba fruit.

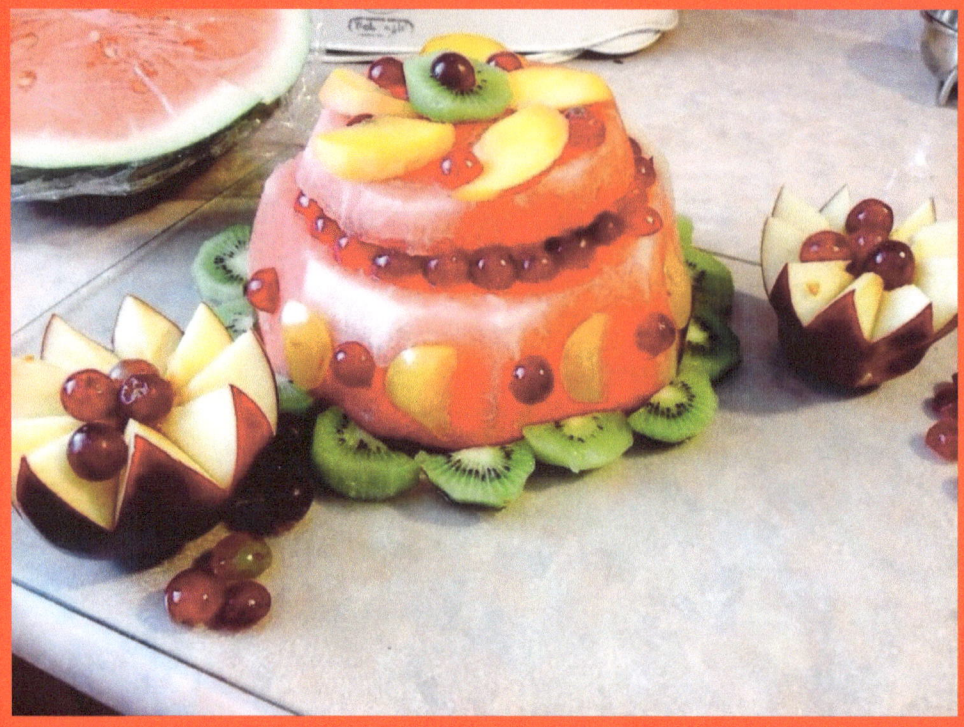

I love to eat more fruits when my mom makes fruit cake!

YUM YUM IN MY TUM!

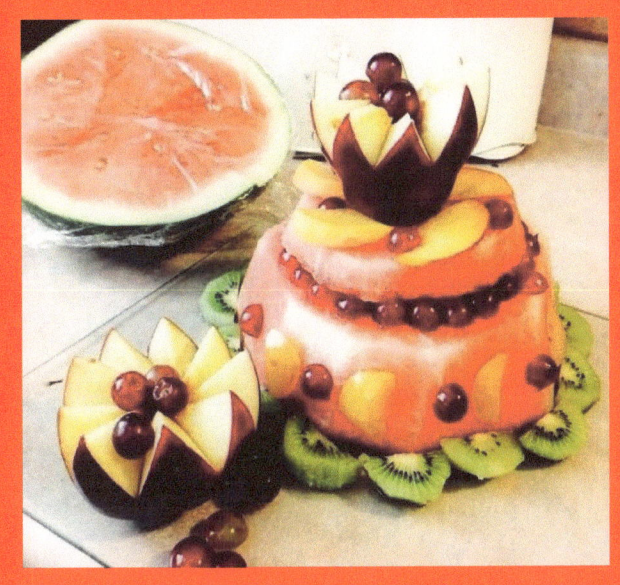

This is for you!

A delicious watermelon fruit cake! Enjoy....

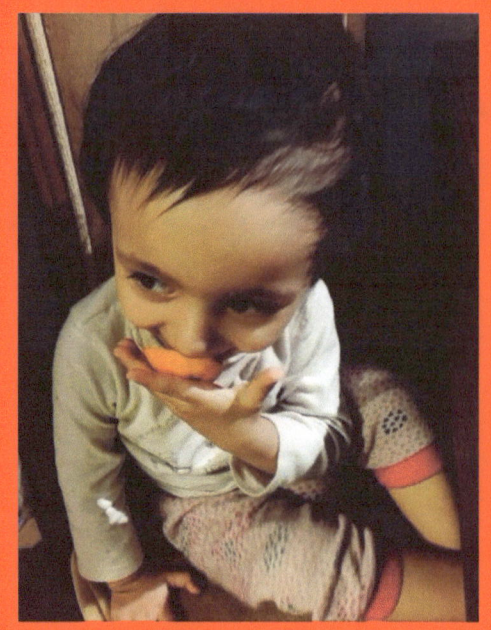

......even baby loves to eat fruit.

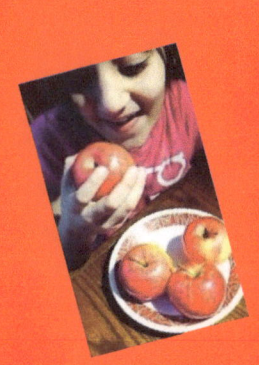
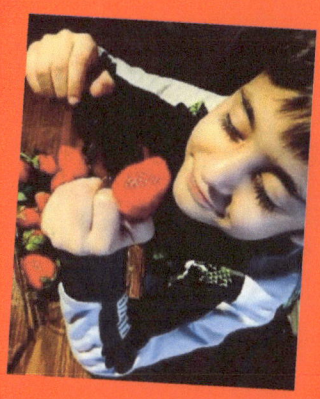
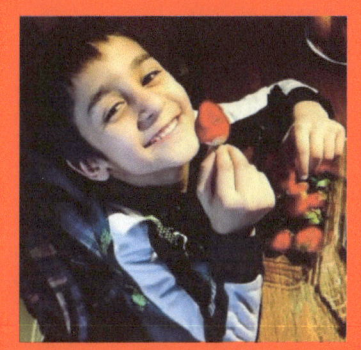

Would you like to eat some FRUIT?

Now it's your turn... ask an adult to give you your favorite fruit and let's have a fruit eating party! Yayyyy.........
and we can try one fruit or smoothie every single day! Promise??...
Thank you!

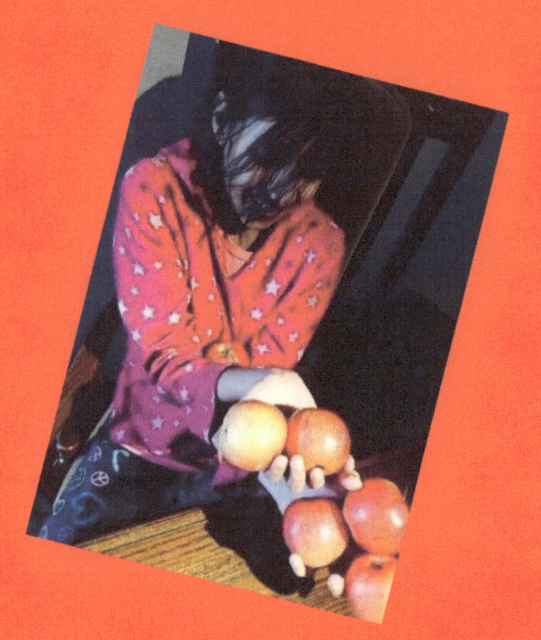

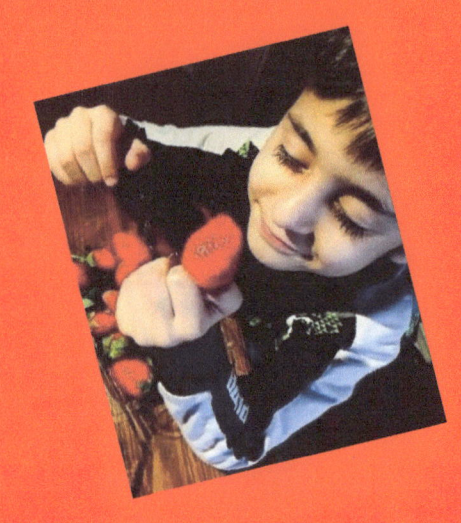

- **DID YOU ENJOY MY BOOK? I WOULD LOVE A REVIEW! PLEASE GIVE ME YOUR HONEST FEEDBACK ON AMAZON!**

- **LOVE THE BOOK AND WANT TO READ MORE? CHECK OUT MY NEW BOOKS WWW.NABILAKIYANI.COM**

- **HIRE ME TO SPEAK, COACH, TRAIN!**
- **HIRE NABILA KIYANI TO SPEAK AT YOUR NEXT EVENT!**

NABILA HAS BEEN SPEAKING TO GROUPS AND ORGANIZATIONS FOR THE PAST 5 YEARS. SHE'S AN EXPERT ON HEALTH COACHING AND MOTIVATIONAL SPEAKER AND HAS HELPED COUNTLESS CLIENTS ACHIEVE THEIR HEALTHIEST GLOW. AUTHOR OF "I LOVE YUMMY FRUITS", NABILA BELIEVES BEAUTY AND HEALTHY EATING HABITS STARTS FROM WITHIN, SO SHE FOLLOWS AN A-Z PROTOCOL TO HELP CLIENTS BECOME HEALTHY EATERS AND RADIANT FROM THE INSIDE OUT. SHE HAS SERVED AS A KEYNOTE FOR MANY ORGANIZATIONS, INCLUDING THE KIP ACADEMY CANADA

FOR MORE INFORMATION OR TO HIRE NABILA FOR YOUR NEXT KEYNOTE, EMAIL NKTYANI@MSN.COM OR CALL 1-(647) 767-5033

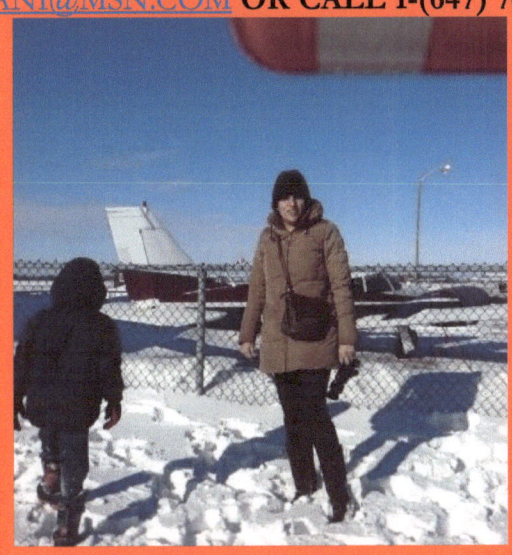

32

==Finally- A book on Fruits from A to Z that helps Parents and Teachers to teach the names of fruits from A – Z rather than vegetable names==.

==Do you know the names of fruits from A to Z?==

==Do you want your child to learn the names of fruits from A to Z?==

==Do you want to read a simple book which has alphabetical fruit names? Instead of Vegetables names?==

Nabila Kiyani, Airplane Pilot, Certified Health Coach, Author, Motivational Speaker and Montessori Directress, can show you a better way for your child to learn the names of fruits in an alphabetical order. She goes down to child's level to understand how a child learns and love to eat healthy.

You'll learn How to Do the following:

❖ Treat your child with healthy sweet fruit alternative to combat Junk food craving.
❖ Learn the names of fruits from around the world.
❖ Increase your child's vocabulary on fruits and
❖ Indirectly encourage your child to live a healthy life style.

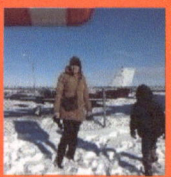

Nabila Kiyani received her training from the Institute for Integrative Nutrition, Algonquin Flight Center and Airline. Nabila works with busy individuals who are ready to take their health to next level. Clients describe her as "inspiring" and "motivating." For more information: Email: nkiyani@msn.com or visit www.aviationmylife.com www.Iloveyummyfruits.com